Sirtfood Diet Meal Plan for Women

A 21-Day Meal Plan and Recipes to Activate Your Body's Natural Weight Management and Health Support System to Lose Weight.

Emilie Dibbert

Copyright © 2024 by Emilie Dibbert

Table of Contents

Introduction

The Sirtfood Diet is a two-phase plan designed to promote weight loss and improve overall health by incorporating sirtuin-activating foods, or "sirtfoods," into your diet. Sirtuins are a group of proteins found in the body that play a role in various cellular processes, including metabolism, inflammation, and lifespan regulation.

The core concept of the Sirtfood Diet lies in activating these sirtuins through specific dietary choices. Proponents of the diet claim that consuming sirtfoods can mimic the effects of calorie restriction and exercise, potentially leading to:

- Increased fat burning: Sirtuins are believed to influence how the body uses fuel for energy, potentially promoting the burning of fat stores.
- Improved cellular health: Sirtuins may enhance cellular repair mechanisms and protect cells from damage.
- Boosted metabolism: Activation of sirtuins might lead to a slight increase in metabolic rate, promoting more calorie burning at rest.
- Reduced inflammation: Sirtuins are thought to have anti-inflammatory properties, potentially contributing to overall health benefits.

The Sirtfood Diet is structured in two distinct phases, each with its own set of guidelines and goals:

- Phase 1: The Activation Phase (7 Days): This initial phase focuses on jump-starting weight loss through a combination of calorie restriction and sirtfood-rich meals. It typically involves consuming green juices and sirtfood-based meals, resulting in a daily calorie intake of around 1000-1200 calories.
- Phase 2: The Maintenance Phase (14 Days and Beyond): This phase aims to establish healthy eating habits for long-term weight management and overall health. It allows for a more balanced and varied diet while still incorporating sirtfoods. Calorie intake increases to around 1500-1800 calories per day.

The Sirtfood Diet also emphasizes the importance of specific sirtfood-rich ingredients like green vegetables, berries, dark chocolate (at least 70% cocoa), and green tea. By incorporating these foods regularly, the diet aims to activate sirtuins and promote the potential health benefits listed above.

How Does the Sirtfood Diet Work for Women?

The Sirtfood Diet can be a potentially effective weight loss strategy for women, but it's crucial to consider the unique hormonal and metabolic factors that influence their bodies. Here's a breakdown of how the Sirtfood Diet might impact women and how to optimize its effectiveness:

Hormonal Fluctuations:

Estrogen and progesterone: These sex hormones play a significant role in regulating appetite, fat storage, and metabolism. Fluctuations throughout the menstrual cycle can affect weight loss efforts.

The Sirtfood Diet can be beneficial by promoting satiety with sirtfoods rich in fiber and healthy fats, potentially helping women manage cravings associated with hormonal changes.

Thyroid function: The thyroid gland produces hormones that regulate metabolism. Conditions like hypothyroidism can make weight loss more challenging.

The Sirtfood Diet, with its focus on calorie reduction and nutrient-dense sirtfoods, can support healthy thyroid function, potentially improving metabolism in some women.

Metabolic Differences:

Muscle mass: Women generally have less muscle mass compared to men. Muscle burns more calories at rest, so women may have a slightly slower metabolism.

The Sirtfood Diet, when combined with regular exercise, can help women build and maintain muscle mass, leading to a more efficient metabolism.

Body fat distribution: Women tend to store more body fat in the hips and thighs compared to men.

While the Sirtfood Diet promotes overall weight loss, it may not specifically target these areas. Exercise strategies targeting these areas can be incorporated alongside the diet.

Optimizing the Sirtfood Diet for Women:

Focus on Nutrient Density: Sirtfoods are rich in vitamins, minerals, and antioxidants, which are especially important for women's health. Prioritize a variety of sirtfoods to ensure a balanced intake of these essential nutrients.

Mindful Eating: The Sirtfood Diet can be restrictive, particularly in Phase 1. Practice mindful eating to avoid overeating or feeling deprived. Focus on savoring food and listening to your body's hunger cues.

Strength Training: Include strength training exercises alongside the Sirtfood Diet. Building muscle mass can boost metabolism and help with weight management in the long run.

Hormonal Awareness: Be mindful of how your hormones might affect your weight loss journey. Track your menstrual cycle and adjust your calorie intake or exercise routine as needed.

Listen to Your Body: Pay attention to your energy levels and adjust the diet accordingly. If you experience extreme fatigue or feel overly restricted, consult a registered dietitian for personalized guidance.

Understanding Sirtuins and Their Benefits

Sirtuins are a group of enzymes found within the cells of our bodies. They belong to a class of proteins known as protein deacetylases, meaning they remove acetyl groups from other proteins. This seemingly simple process has a profound impact on various cellular functions, influencing how our bodies function at a fundamental level.

Benefits of Sirtuins:

Research suggests that sirtuins play a crucial role in promoting healthy aging and overall well-being. Here's a glimpse into some of the potential benefits associated with sirtuin activity:

Cellular Health and Repair: Sirtuins are believed to support DNA repair mechanisms, potentially protecting cells from damage and promoting healthy aging.

Increased Longevity: Studies in various organisms have linked sirtuin activation to extended lifespan. While the exact mechanisms in humans are still being explored, the connection is promising.

Enhanced Metabolism: Sirtuins may influence how the body uses fuel for energy, potentially promoting fat burning and a more efficient metabolism.

Improved Insulin Sensitivity: Sirtuins might play a role in regulating blood sugar levels by enhancing insulin sensitivity, potentially benefiting those with prediabetes or type 2 diabetes.

Anti-inflammatory Properties: Research suggests that sirtuins have anti-inflammatory effects, which can contribute to overall health and reduce the risk of chronic diseases.

What to Expect from the Sirtfood Diet

Weight Loss Potential:

The Sirtfood Diet is designed to promote weight loss, particularly in the initial phase with its calorie restriction and focus on sirtfoods. Here's what you might experience:

- Rapid Weight Loss in Phase 1: The first week typically involves a significant reduction in calorie intake, potentially leading to rapid weight loss (around 7 pounds). However, it's important to remember that some of this weight loss might be water weight.

- Gradual Weight Loss in Phase 2: As the diet progresses to Phase 2, calorie intake increases and weight loss becomes more gradual and sustainable.

Potential Health Benefits:

Beyond weight loss, the Sirtfood Diet, with its emphasis on sirtfoods rich in vitamins, minerals, and antioxidants, might offer additional health benefits:

- Improved Blood Sugar Control: Sirtuins may enhance insulin sensitivity, potentially benefiting those with prediabetes or type 2 diabetes by promoting better blood sugar regulation.

- Reduced Inflammation: The anti-inflammatory properties of sirtuins could contribute to a decreased risk of chronic diseases associated with inflammation.

- Enhanced Cellular Health: Sirtuin activation might support DNA repair and cellular health, potentially promoting healthy aging.

Chapter 1: The Two Phases of the Sirtfood Diet

Phase 1 of the Sirtfood Diet serves as the foundation, aiming to jumpstart your weight loss by activating sirtuins and promoting rapid weight loss.

Structure and Duration:

- Duration: Phase 1 lasts for seven days.
- Focus: This phase emphasizes calorie restriction and incorporating sirtfoods into your diet to activate sirtuins.

Daily Routine:

Green Juices: You'll consume three green sirtfood juices throughout the day, spaced evenly. These juices are packed with sirtfoods and provide essential vitamins and minerals.

Sirtfood Meal: One sirtfood-rich meal is included each day. This meal should be filling but adhere to the calorie restrictions of Phase 1.

Calorie Intake:

Calorie Range: The daily calorie intake in Phase 1 typically falls between 1000 and 1200 calories. This calorie restriction is designed to trigger the body's response similar to calorie restriction, potentially promoting sirtuin activation.

Sample Meal Plans:

Day 1:

Green Juice 1: Kale, spinach, celery, apple, green tea, lemon juice

Green Juice 2: Green tea, parsley, arugula, strawberries, lemon juice

Green Juice 3: Buckwheat, kale, matcha green tea, berries, almond milk

Sirtfood Meal: Shrimp stir-fry with buckwheat noodles and vegetables (around 400-500 calories)

Day 2:

Green Juice (repeat any from Day 1): Choose two of your favorites from Day 1

Green Juice (new option): Kale, celery, apple, ginger, parsley, lemon juice

Sirtfood Meal: Miso-glazed tofu with roasted vegetables and quinoa (around 400-500 calories)

Day 3:

Green Juice (repeat any from Day 1 or 2): Choose one from previous days

Green Juice (new option): Spinach, romaine lettuce, celery, pear, green tea, lemon juice

Sirtfood Meal: Sirtfood salad with mixed greens, berries, walnuts, and a sirtfood dressing (around 400-500 calories)

Green Juice Recipes

Green juices are a cornerstone of Phase 1 in the Sirtfood Diet. These nutrient-packed beverages are rich in sirtfoods and provide essential vitamins, minerals, and antioxidants to support your weight loss goals and overall health.

Green Juice Basics:

Base: Always start with a leafy green base like kale, spinach, or romaine lettuce. These greens provide a foundation of vitamins, minerals, and fiber.

Sirtfood Powerhouses: Incorporate a variety of sirtfoods into your juices. Popular choices include berries (strawberries, blueberries, raspberries), apples, celery, parsley, and green tea.

Liquids: Use water for a lighter juice or unsweetened almond milk for a creamier texture.

Flavor Boosters: For an extra flavor kick, consider adding a squeeze of lemon or lime juice, a small piece of ginger, or a pinch of matcha green tea.

Sweeteners (Optional): While the sweetness from fruits in the juice is generally enough, you can add a touch of natural sweetener like stevia if desired. However, use sparingly as Phase 1 emphasizes calorie restriction.

Green Juice Recipes:

1. Berry Blast:

Ingredients:

1 cup kale

1/2 cup spinach

1/2 cup mixed berries (strawberries, blueberries, raspberries)

1 apple (cored)

1/2 inch ginger (peeled)

1 cup water

1/2 lemon, juiced (optional)

2. Tropical Twist:

Ingredients:

1 cup romaine lettuce

1/2 cup green tea (brewed and cooled)

1/2 cup pineapple (fresh or frozen)

1/4 cup celery

1/4 cup parsley

1/2 cup unsweetened almond milk

Pinch of matcha green tea (optional)

3. Green Goddess:

Ingredients:

1 cup baby kale

1/2 cup cucumber (peeled)

1/2 avocado (peeled and pitted)

1/2 cup green grapes

1/4 cup celery

1/4 cup parsley

1 cup water

Squeeze of lime juice (optional)

4. Spicy Sunrise:

Ingredients:

1 cup spinach

1/2 cup cantaloupe (flesh only)

1/4 cup celery

1/4 cup cilantro

1/2 inch ginger (peeled)

1/4 jalapeno pepper (seeded, optional for extra spice)

1 cup water

1/2 lemon, juiced

5. Matcha Mania:

Ingredients:

1 cup arugula

1/2 cup green tea (brewed and cooled)

1/2 cup pear (cored)

1/4 cup celery

1/4 cup mint leaves

1/2 cup unsweetened almond milk

1 tsp matcha green tea

Sirtfood-Rich Meal Options

Phase 1 of the Sirtfood Diet emphasizes sirtfood-rich meals alongside green juices to activate sirtuins and promote weight loss.

Sirtfood Meal Essentials:

Focus on Sirtfoods: Prioritize incorporating a variety of sirtfoods into your meals. Refer to the sirtfood list in Part 2 of this book for inspiration.

Calorie Control: Keep your meals within the Phase 1 calorie range (around 400-500 calories per meal).

Nutrient Balance: Aim for a balanced meal with sirtfoods from different categories like leafy greens, fruits, whole grains, and lean proteins.

Flavor and Variety: Experiment with different sirtfood combinations to keep your meals exciting and enjoyable throughout Phase 1.

Sample Sirtfood Meals for Phase 1:

Breakfast (around 300-350 calories):

- Sirtfood Oatmeal: Prepare oatmeal with water or unsweetened almond milk, top with berries, a sprinkle of walnuts, and a drizzle of dark chocolate sauce (at least 70% cocoa).

- Sirtfood Smoothie Bowl: Blend together a handful of spinach, half a banana, some strawberries, and unsweetened almond milk. Pour into a bowl and top with chopped walnuts, chia seeds, and a sprinkle of dark chocolate shavings.

- Sirtfood Yogurt Parfait: Layer a serving of plain Greek yogurt with chopped apple, berries, and a sprinkle of ground cinnamon.

Lunch (around 350-400 calories):

- Sirtfood Salad: Create a salad base with mixed greens, add chopped kale, sliced strawberries, walnuts, and top with a sirtfood dressing made with olive oil, lemon juice, and a touch of Dijon mustard.

- Sirtfood Soup: Prepare a light soup with vegetable broth, chopped kale, lentils, and a dash of turmeric. Enjoy with a side of whole-wheat crackers.

- Sirtfood Buddha Bowl: Combine cooked quinoa, roasted chickpeas, chopped vegetables (broccoli, carrots), and a drizzle of tahini sauce.

Dinner (around 400-450 calories):

- Sirtfood Stir-Fry: Stir-fry tofu or shrimp with a medley of sirtfoods like broccoli, bell peppers, and onions. Serve over buckwheat noodles or quinoa.
- Sirtfood Salmon with Roasted Vegetables: Bake salmon with a squeeze of lemon juice and herbs. Roast asparagus and cherry tomatoes on the side for a complete meal.
- Sirtfood Turkey Chili: Prepare a chili with ground turkey, chopped tomatoes, kidney beans, and a variety of sirtfood vegetables like bell peppers, onions, and celery.

Phase 2: The Maintenance Phase

Phase 1 of the Sirtfood Diet provides a kickstart for weight loss through calorie restriction and sirtuin activation. Phase 2, however, is where the emphasis shifts towards building sustainable healthy eating habits for long-term success.

Structure and Duration:

- Duration: Phase 2 can last for as long as you desire. The goal is to establish healthy eating patterns that become a way of life.
- Focus: This phase emphasizes incorporating sirtfoods into a balanced diet with a moderate increase in calorie intake compared to Phase 1.

Building Healthy Habits:

Phase 2 encourages a shift in mindset from short-term weight loss to long-term health and well-being. Here are some key principles to focus on:

- Portion Control: Learn to practice mindful eating and portion control to maintain a healthy weight.
- Balanced Meals: Strive for balanced meals that include sirtfoods from different categories like vegetables, fruits, whole grains, and lean protein sources.

- Variety is Key: Include a diverse range of sirtfoods in your diet to ensure you receive a broad spectrum of essential nutrients.
- Cook More Often: Preparing meals at home allows you to control ingredients and portion sizes.
- Stay Hydrated: Drinking plenty of water throughout the day is crucial for overall health and supports healthy eating habits.
- Regular Exercise: Combine your healthy eating habits with regular physical activity for optimal weight management and well-being.

Calorie Intake in Phase 2:

Increased Calorie Range: Phase 2 allows for a more moderate calorie intake, typically ranging from 1500 to 1800 calories per day. This increase provides more energy for daily activities and helps sustain weight loss.

Maintaining Sirtuin Activation:

While not as restrictive as Phase 1, Phase 2 still encourages incorporating sirtfoods into your diet. Here are ways to maintain sirtuin activation:

- Include Sirtfoods in Every Meal: Aim to have at least one sirtfood in each meal or snack.

- Maintain a Green Juice Habit: While not mandatory, continuing to enjoy a green juice occasionally can provide a good source of sirtfoods and nutrients.

- Explore New Sirtfood Recipes: Experiment with new recipes to keep your meals exciting and maintain motivation during Phase 2.

Sample Meal Plans for Phase 2:

Breakfast (around 400-450 calories):

- Sirtfood Pancakes: Prepare pancakes using buckwheat flour, top with berries and a drizzle of maple syrup.

- Sirtfood Scramble: Scramble eggs with chopped vegetables like spinach and tomatoes, serve with a slice of whole-wheat toast.

- Sirtfood Yogurt Bowl: Layer Greek yogurt with granola, chopped apple, berries, and a sprinkle of chia seeds.

Lunch (around 500-550 calories):

- Sirtfood Salad with Grilled Chicken: Combine mixed greens with quinoa, grilled chicken breast, sliced avocado, and a sirtfood dressing.

- Sirtfood Lentil Soup: Enjoy a bowl of lentil soup with chopped vegetables and a side salad.

- Sirtfood Buddha Bowl with Tofu: Combine brown rice, roasted vegetables, crumbled tofu, and a drizzle of tahini sauce.

Dinner (around 550-600 calories):

- Sirtfood Salmon with Roasted Brussels Sprouts: Bake salmon with lemon and herbs, pair it with roasted Brussels sprouts and quinoa.
- Sirtfood Turkey Chili with Whole-Wheat Bread: Enjoy a bowl of turkey chili with a slice of whole-wheat bread.
- Sirtfood Stir-Fry with Shrimp and Vegetables: Stir-fry shrimp with a variety of sirtfoods like broccoli, bell peppers, and onions. Serve over brown rice.

Building Balanced Meals with Sirtfoods

Phase 2 of the Sirtfood Diet marks a shift towards establishing healthy eating habits for long-term weight management.

Planning Balanced Meals:

Phase 2 encourages balanced meals that incorporate sirtfoods from various categories to ensure a well-rounded intake of nutrients. Here's a breakdown of key components to consider:

- Sirtfood Vegetables: Vegetables are a cornerstone of healthy eating and provide essential vitamins, minerals, and fiber. Aim for a variety of sirtfood vegetables like kale, spinach, arugula, broccoli, onions, and bell peppers.
- Sirtfood Fruits: Fruits add sweetness, vitamins, and antioxidants to your meals. Berries (blueberries,

strawberries, raspberries), apples, pears, and citrus fruits are all excellent sirtfood choices.

- Whole Grains: Opt for whole grains like brown rice, quinoa, buckwheat, and whole-wheat bread for sustained energy and fiber.

- Lean Protein Sources: Include lean protein sources like chicken breast, fish, tofu, lentils, or beans to support muscle mass and satiety.

- Healthy Fats: Don't shy away from healthy fats like those found in olive oil, avocado, nuts, and seeds. These fats contribute to satiety and support nutrient absorption.

Sample Recipes for Balanced Phase 2 Meals:

Sirtfood Breakfast Bowl (around 400 calories):

Ingredients:

- 1/2 cup cooked quinoa
- 1/2 cup chopped kale
- 1/4 cup blueberries
- 1/4 cup sliced almonds
- 1/4 cup plain Greek yogurt
- 1 tablespoon chia seeds
- Drizzle of honey (optional)

Instructions:

1. Combine cooked quinoa, kale, blueberries, and almonds in a bowl.

2. Top with Greek yogurt and chia seeds.

3. Drizzle with honey for a touch of sweetness (optional).

Sirtfood Chicken Salad Sandwich (around 500 calories):

Ingredients:

- 2 slices whole-wheat bread
- 4 ounces grilled chicken breast, sliced
- 1/2 cup mixed greens
- 1/4 cup chopped tomato
- 1/4 cup sliced avocado
- 2 tablespoons sirtfood dressing (olive oil, lemon juice, spices)

Instructions:

1. Toast whole-wheat bread slices.

2. Layer chicken breast, mixed greens, tomato, and avocado on one bread slice.

3. Drizzle with sirtfood dressing and top with the other bread slice.

Sirtfood Salmon with Roasted Vegetables (around 600 calories):

Ingredients:

- 4 ounces salmon fillet
- 1 tablespoon olive oil
- 1/2 lemon, juiced
- 1 cup broccoli florets
- 1 cup Brussels sprouts, halved
- 1/2 cup quinoa
- Salt and pepper to taste

Instructions:

1. Preheat oven to 400°F (200°C).

2. Toss broccoli and Brussels sprouts with olive oil, salt, and pepper. Spread on a baking sheet and roast for 20 minutes.

3. Season salmon with salt, pepper, and lemon juice. Bake alongside vegetables for 15-20 minutes, or until cooked through.

4. Cook quinoa according to package instructions.

5. Serve salmon with roasted vegetables and cooked quinoa.

Meal Planning Strategies:

- Plan Your Week: Dedicate time each week to plan your meals and create a grocery list to stay on track with your sirtfood choices.
- Prep in Advance: Wash and chop vegetables, cook grains in advance, or prepare sirtfood snacks like sliced apples with almond butter to save time during busy days.
- Cook More Often: Cooking meals at home allows you to control ingredients, portion sizes, and incorporate a variety of sirtfoods.
- Leftovers are Your Friend: Cook larger batches for leftovers to ensure you have healthy meals readily available throughout the week.
- Don't Be Afraid to Snack: Include sirtfood-rich snacks like berries, nuts, or a small green juice to curb cravings and prevent overeating at meals.

Maintaining Weight Loss and Healthy Habits

The Sirtfood Diet can be a helpful tool for jumpstarting weight loss and establishing healthy habits. However, long-term weight management and overall well-being require a more holistic approach.

Sustainable Lifestyle Changes:

The key to lasting success lies in shifting your mindset from short-term dieting to creating sustainable lifestyle changes. Here are some key areas to focus on:

- Mindful Eating: Practice mindful eating habits to develop a healthy relationship with food. Pay attention to hunger and fullness cues, and avoid emotional eating.
- Portion Control: Continue to practice mindful portion control to maintain a healthy calorie intake and prevent weight regain.
- Balanced Meals: Strive for balanced meals that incorporate whole grains, lean protein, healthy fats, fruits, and vegetables to ensure your body receives the nutrients it needs.
- Variety is Key: Include a diverse range of sirtfoods and other healthy foods in your diet to maintain a balanced intake of nutrients and keep your meals interesting.
- Planning and Preparation: Plan your meals and snacks for the week, and prepare healthy options in advance to avoid unhealthy choices when pressed for time.
- Cook More Often: Cooking meals at home allows you to control ingredients, portion sizes, and sodium content.
- Stay Hydrated: Drinking plenty of water throughout the day is crucial for overall health, supports digestion, and helps you feel full.

- **Regular Exercise:** Make physical activity a regular part of your life. Aim for at least 30 minutes of moderate-intensity exercise most days of the week. Exercise helps burn calories, build muscle mass, and improves overall health.

- **Quality Sleep:** Prioritize quality sleep for at least 7-8 hours each night. Adequate sleep regulates hormones that influence hunger and satiety, and can impact your weight management efforts.

- **Manage Stress:** Chronic stress can contribute to weight gain. Find healthy ways to manage stress, such as yoga, meditation, or spending time in nature.

Chapter 2: Top Sirtfoods for Women

Fruits

Women have unique nutritional needs throughout their life stages. Sirtfoods can be valuable allies in supporting these needs. Here's how some sirtfood fruits can be particularly beneficial for women:

- Hormonal Balance: Certain sirtfoods may support hormonal health, potentially aiding with menstrual regularity and menopausal symptoms.
- Bone Health: Sirtuins may play a role in bone health, and sirtfood fruits rich in calcium and vitamin K can be especially helpful.
- Immune System Function: Sirtfoods rich in antioxidants can contribute to a strong immune system, important for overall well-being.
- Skin Health: Antioxidants in sirtfood fruits can help protect against skin damage and promote a healthy glow.

Top Sirtfood Fruits for Women:

1. Berries (Blueberries, Strawberries, Raspberries):

Benefits: These antioxidant powerhouses are packed with vitamins, minerals, and fiber. They may contribute to hormonal balance, heart health, and healthy aging.

2. Apples:

Benefits: Rich in fiber and quercetin, an antioxidant that may support bone health and heart health.

3. Citrus Fruits (Grapefruits, Oranges):

Benefits: Excellent source of vitamin C, crucial for immune function and collagen production for healthy skin.

4. Pomegranates:

Benefits: Rich in antioxidants with anti-inflammatory properties that may benefit heart health and potentially hormonal health.

5. Dates:

Benefits: A good source of natural sugars, fiber, and minerals like iron, which can be especially important during menstruation and pregnancy.

Enjoy These Sirtfood Fruits:

- Include sirtfood fruits in your green juices for a concentrated nutrient boost.
- Snack on fresh sirtfood fruits throughout the day to curb cravings and provide sustained energy.
- Add sirtfood fruits to yogurt parfaits, smoothies, or oatmeal for a delicious and nutritious breakfast.
- Experiment with sirtfood fruits in salads or homemade desserts for a healthy twist.

Vegetables

Vegetables provide essential vitamins, minerals, fiber, and antioxidants that contribute significantly to women's health throughout various life stages. Here's how some sirtfood vegetables can be particularly beneficial:

- Hormonal Health: Certain sirtfoods may support hormonal balance, potentially aiding with menstrual regularity and menopausal symptoms.
- Bone Health: Sirtuins may play a role in bone health, and sirtfood vegetables rich in calcium and vitamin K can be especially helpful.
- Cellular Health: Antioxidant-rich sirtfood vegetables can help protect cells from damage and promote overall well-being.
- Weight Management: Vegetables are low in calories and high in fiber, promoting satiety and aiding in weight management.

Top Sirtfood Vegetables for Women:

1. Cruciferous Vegetables (Kale, Broccoli, Brussels Sprouts):

Benefits: Rich in sulforaphane, a compound with potential benefits for hormonal health and detoxification.

2. Leafy Greens (Spinach, Arugula, Romaine Lettuce):

Benefits: Excellent source of vitamins, minerals, and antioxidants that support bone health, immune function, and skin health.

3. Green Beans:

Benefits: A good source of fiber and folate, important for cell health and fetal development during pregnancy.

4. Onions and Garlic:

Benefits: Contain prebiotics that support gut health, which can influence hormonal balance and overall well-being.

5. Celery:

Benefits: High in water content and low in calories, promoting hydration and aiding in weight management.

Get Creative with Sirtfood Vegetables:

Roast sirtfood vegetables with olive oil and herbs for a flavorful side dish.

Add chopped sirtfood vegetables to omelets, frittatas, or stir-fries for a nutrient boost.

Use sirtfood vegetables to create healthy soups and stews.

Enjoy sirtfood vegetables with hummus or a healthy dip for a satisfying snack.

Blend sirtfood vegetables into green juices or smoothies for a concentrated dose of nutrients.

Grains

Grains offer a variety of health benefits, and sirtfood grains can be especially valuable for women. Here's how incorporating sirtfood grains can support your well-being:

- Hormonal Health: Whole grains may help regulate blood sugar levels, which can indirectly influence hormonal balance.

- Energy Levels: Sirtfood grains are complex carbohydrates, providing sustained energy throughout the day.

- Digestive Health: Fiber in whole grains promotes gut health, which can positively impact overall health and potentially hormonal balance.

- Heart Health: Whole grains are a good source of fiber and may help lower cholesterol levels, contributing to heart health.

Top Sirtfood Grains for Women:

1. Buckwheat:

Benefits: A gluten-free pseudo-grain rich in protein and fiber. Buckwheat may help manage blood sugar and promote satiety.

2. Quinoa:

Benefits: A complete protein source containing all essential amino acids. Quinoa is also high in fiber and iron, important for women, particularly during menstruation and pregnancy.

3. Whole-Wheat Bread:

Benefits: A good source of fiber and complex carbohydrates, providing sustained energy and promoting gut health. Choose whole-wheat bread over refined options.

4. Oats:

Benefits: A heart-healthy grain rich in fiber and beta-glucans, which may help regulate blood sugar and cholesterol levels. Oats are also a good source of iron and can be a filling breakfast option.

5. Brown Rice:

Benefits: A source of complex carbohydrates and fiber, brown rice offers sustained energy and can contribute to digestive health.

Get the Most Out of Sirtfood Grains:

- Enjoy sirtfood grains like rolled oats or quinoa for breakfast with berries and nuts for added nutrients.
- Use cooked quinoa or brown rice as a base for bowls with roasted vegetables, lean protein, and a sirtfood dressing.
- Add whole-wheat bread to sandwiches filled with sirtfood vegetables and lean protein sources.
- Explore recipes for sirtfood grain salads or grain bowls for a satisfying and nutritious lunch option.

Legumes

Legumes are a nutritional powerhouse, providing protein, fiber, vitamins, and minerals that contribute significantly to women's health throughout various life stages. Here's a closer look at how sirtfood legumes can be particularly beneficial:

- Hormonal Health: Plant-based protein in legumes may help regulate blood sugar levels, which can indirectly influence hormonal balance.
- Bone Health: Legumes are a good source of plant-based calcium and iron, both crucial for maintaining strong bones, especially important during pregnancy and menopause.
- Energy Levels: Legumes are a complex carbohydrate source, providing sustained energy and promoting satiety.
- Digestive Health: Fiber in legumes supports gut health, which can positively impact overall health and potentially hormonal balance.

Top Sirtfood Legumes for Women:

1. Lentils:

Benefits: Rich in protein, fiber, iron, and folate. Lentils are a versatile ingredient for soups, stews, salads, and vegetarian burgers.

2. Chickpeas (Garbanzo Beans):

Benefits: A good source of protein, fiber, folate, and iron. Chickpeas are perfect for hummus, falafel, salads, and curries.

3. Edamame (Soybeans):

Benefits: A complete protein source containing all essential amino acids. Edamame is also rich in isoflavones, which have a similar structure to estrogen and may offer benefits during menopause.

4. Peas (Snap Peas, Green Peas):

Benefits: A good source of protein, fiber, vitamin K, and iron. Peas are a versatile addition to stir-fries, salads, and soups.

5. Black Beans:

Benefits: Rich in protein, fiber, folate, and antioxidants. Black beans are a staple in many cuisines and can be used in soups, salads, tacos, and dips.

Unlocking the Potential of Sirtfood Legumes:

- Enjoy a bowl of lentil soup with whole-wheat bread for a satisfying and nutritious lunch.
- Toss cooked chickpeas or black beans into a salad for added protein and fiber.
- Make a batch of homemade hummus with chickpeas, tahini, olive oil, and lemon juice for a healthy dip or spread.

- Experiment with vegetarian burgers or meatballs made with lentils, chickpeas, or black beans.
- Add edamame pods to stir-fries or enjoy them as a healthy snack with a sprinkle of sea salt.

Healthy Fats

Including healthy fats in your diet is essential for women's health across various life stages. Here's how incorporating sirtfood healthy fats can support your well-being:

- Hormonal Health: Healthy fats are necessary for hormone production and regulation, potentially aiding with menstrual regularity and menopausal symptoms.
- Brain Health: Healthy fats are essential for cognitive function and may help protect against cognitive decline.
- Heart Health: Healthy fats can help lower bad cholesterol (LDL) levels and improve heart health.
- Nutrient Absorption: Certain vitamins are fat-soluble, and healthy fats are needed for their proper absorption.
- Skin and Hair Health: Healthy fats contribute to healthy, glowing skin and promote strong hair.

Top Sirtfood Healthy Fats for Women:

1. Olive Oil:

Benefits: Rich in monounsaturated fats and antioxidants with anti-inflammatory properties. Olive oil may benefit heart health and cognitive function.

2. Avocados:

Benefits: A good source of monounsaturated fats, fiber, and potassium. Avocados can promote satiety and support heart health.

3. Nuts and Seeds (Almonds, Walnuts, Chia Seeds):

Benefits: A source of healthy fats, protein, fiber, vitamins, and minerals. Nuts and seeds contribute to satiety, heart health, and gut health.

4. Fatty Fish (Salmon, Sardines, Mackerel):

Benefits: Rich in omega-3 fatty acids, essential for brain health, heart health, and potentially reducing inflammation.

5. Dark Chocolate (at least 70% cocoa):

Benefits: Contains moderate amounts of healthy fats and flavanols, antioxidants that may benefit heart health and cognitive function. Enjoy in moderation due to sugar content.

Adding Sirtfood Healthy Fats to Your Diet:

- Drizzle olive oil on salads, roasted vegetables, or whole grains.

- Include half an avocado in your lunch salad or breakfast toast for added creaminess and healthy fats.

- Enjoy a handful of nuts or seeds as a healthy snack, or add them to yogurt parfaits or oatmeal.

- Aim for 2-3 servings of fatty fish per week for a good source of omega-3 fatty acids.

- Enjoy a small square of dark chocolate after dinner for a satisfying treat with a dose of antioxidants.

Beverages

Staying hydrated is crucial for various bodily functions and overall well-being. Sirtfood beverages can offer additional benefits beyond hydration, particularly for women:

- Hormonal Health: Certain beverages may support hormonal balance, potentially aiding with menstrual regularity and menopausal symptoms.

- Bone Health: Some beverages can contribute to bone health by providing essential minerals like calcium and magnesium.

- Metabolism Boost: Certain beverages may slightly increase metabolism, aiding in weight management.

- Antioxidant Power: Sirtfood beverages rich in antioxidants can help protect cells from damage and promote overall well-being.

Top Sirtfood Beverages for Women:

1. Green Tea:

Benefits: Rich in antioxidants with anti-inflammatory properties. Green tea may support heart health, cognitive function, and potentially hormonal balance.

2. Coffee (in moderation):

Benefits: Contains moderate amounts of caffeine, which can improve alertness and boost metabolism slightly. Coffee also offers antioxidants with potential health benefits.

3. Water with Lemon:

Benefits: Provides essential hydration and supports digestion. Lemon adds a refreshing flavor and may offer a small metabolic boost.

4. Herbal Teas (Peppermint, Hibiscus):

Benefits: Can be naturally caffeine-free and offer various health benefits depending on the specific herb. Peppermint tea may aid digestion, while hibiscus tea may have mild blood pressure-lowering properties.

5. Sirtfood Green Juice:

Benefits: A concentrated source of sirtfoods and nutrients from vegetables and fruits. Green juices can be a convenient way to incorporate a variety of sirtfoods into your diet and potentially support detoxification.

Enjoying Sirtfood Beverages:

- Start your day with a cup of green tea for a refreshing and potentially metabolism-boosting beverage.
- Enjoy a cup of coffee in moderation for a pick-me-up and potential cognitive benefits.
- Sip on water with lemon throughout the day to stay hydrated and support digestion.
- Choose herbal teas based on your needs - peppermint for digestion or hibiscus for a potential blood pressure-lowering effect (consult a doctor if managing blood pressure).
- Include sirtfood green juices occasionally as a way to boost your intake of sirtfoods and nutrients.

Chapter 3: Creating a Sirtfood-Rich Pantry

A well-stocked pantry filled with sirtfoods sets you up for success on your weight management journey. Here's a breakdown of key sirtfood categories to consider:

- Fruits: Berries (blueberries, strawberries, raspberries), apples, citrus fruits (grapefruits, oranges), pomegranates, dates.
- Vegetables: Leafy greens (kale, spinach, arugula), cruciferous vegetables (broccoli, Brussels sprouts), green beans, onions, garlic, celery.
- Grains: Buckwheat, quinoa, whole-wheat bread, oats, brown rice.
- Legumes: Lentils, chickpeas, edamame, peas (snap peas, green peas), black beans.
- Healthy Fats: Olive oil, avocados, nuts and seeds (almonds, walnuts, chia seeds).
- Beverages: Green tea, coffee (in moderation), water with lemon, herbal teas (peppermint, hibiscus).
- Optional: Dark chocolate (at least 70% cocoa) for occasional consumption.

Sirtfood Shopping List:

Fresh Produce:

- Stock up on a variety of fresh sirtfood fruits and vegetables according to your preferences and seasonal availability.
- Consider buying frozen fruits and vegetables for convenience and extended shelf life.

Pantry Staples:

- Purchase whole grains like buckwheat, quinoa, and brown rice in bulk for cost-effectiveness.
- Choose whole-wheat bread over refined options.
- Stock up on dried legumes like lentils, chickpeas, and black beans. Opt for canned options if time is limited, but be mindful of sodium content.
- Healthy fats like olive oil, nuts, and seeds can be purchased in bulk or resealable containers.

Drinks:

- Keep a good supply of green tea, herbal teas, and lemons for water on hand.
- Remember: Adjust this list based on your dietary needs, preferences, and budget.

Storage Tips for Sirtfood Freshness:

- Fruits and Vegetables: Wash and store fruits and vegetables in the crisper drawer of your refrigerator.

- Store leafy greens in a separate container with a damp paper towel to maintain freshness.
- Berries are best stored unwashed until ready to consume.
- Store some fruits like apples at room temperature, while others like berries are best refrigerated.

Grains:

- Keep whole grains like buckwheat, quinoa, and brown rice in airtight containers in a cool, dark pantry.
- Store rolled oats in an airtight container to prevent moisture and potential spoilage.

Legumes:

- Store dried legumes in airtight containers in a cool, dark pantry. Soaked or cooked legumes should be stored in the refrigerator in an airtight container for up to 5 days.

Nuts and Seeds:

- Store nuts and seeds in airtight containers in the refrigerator or freezer to prevent rancidity.

Healthy Fats:

- Store olive oil in a cool, dark pantry away from heat and light.
- Once opened, store avocado oil in the refrigerator.

Beverages:

- Store tea bags in a cool, dark pantry.
- Lemons can be stored at room temperature for a few days or in the crisper drawer of your refrigerator for longer storage.

Chapter 4: Sample 7-Day Meal Plans for Phase 1

Calorie Levels:

- Low Calorie (around 1000 kcal): This plan is suitable for individuals with a lower body weight or minimal physical activity.
- Medium Calorie (around 1200-1500 kcal): This plan caters to a broader range of individuals with moderate activity levels.
- High Calorie (around 1600-1800 kcal): This plan is designed for individuals with a higher body weight or those engaging in regular exercise.

Sample 7-Day Low Calorie Meal Plan (Around 1000 kcal):

Day 1:

- Breakfast: Sirtfood Green Juice (kale, spinach, celery, apple, green tea)
- Lunch: Sirtfood Green Juice (kale, parsley, apple, lemon, matcha)
- Dinner: Grilled Chicken Breast with Kale Salad (olive oil and lemon dressing)

Day 2:

- Breakfast: Sirtfood Green Juice (spinach, celery, pear, ginger)
- Lunch: Sirtfood Green Juice (kale, celery, apple, green tea)
- Dinner: Shrimp Stir-fry with Buckwheat Noodles and Vegetables (broccoli, carrots)

Day 3:

- Breakfast: Sirtfood Green Juice (kale, spinach, strawberries, green tea)
- Lunch: Sirtfood Green Juice (celery, apple, green tea)
- Dinner: Turkey Meatballs with Tomato Sauce and a side of Roasted Brussels Sprouts

Day 4:

- Breakfast: Sirtfood Green Juice (kale, spinach, blueberries, green tea)
- Lunch: Sirtfood Green Juice (celery, apple, lemon)
- Dinner: Salmon with Roasted Vegetables (asparagus, bell peppers)

Day 5:

- Breakfast: Sirtfood Green Juice (spinach, parsley, apple, matcha)
- Lunch: Sirtfood Green Juice (kale, celery, pear, ginger)
- Dinner: Lentil Soup with a side salad (spinach, tomatoes)

Day 6:

- Breakfast: Sirtfood Green Juice (kale, spinach, strawberries, green tea)
- Lunch: Sirtfood Green Juice (celery, apple, lemon)
- Dinner: Chicken Breast with Quinoa Salad (mixed greens, avocado)

Day 7:

- Breakfast: Sirtfood Green Juice (spinach, celery, blueberries, green tea)
- Lunch: Sirtfood Green Juice (kale, apple, green tea)
- Dinner: Tofu Scramble with Vegetables (onions, peppers) and a slice of whole-wheat toast

Sample 7-Day Medium Calorie Meal Plan (Around 1200-1500 kcal):

Day 1:

- Breakfast: Sirtfood Green Juice (kale, spinach, celery, apple, green tea) + a small handful of almonds
- Lunch: Sirtfood Green Juice (kale, parsley, apple, lemon, matcha) + a grilled chicken breast
- Dinner: Grilled Salmon with Roasted Vegetables (asparagus, bell peppers) and a drizzle of olive oil

Day 2:

- Breakfast: Sirtfood Green Juice (spinach, celery, pear, ginger) + ¼ cup rolled oats with berries and a sprinkle of chia seeds
- Lunch: Sirtfood Green Juice (kale, celery, apple, green tea) + a bowl of lentil soup with a slice of whole-wheat bread
- Dinner: Shrimp Stir-fry with Buckwheat Noodles and Vegetables (broccoli, carrots) with a drizzle of sesame oil

Day 3:

- Breakfast: Sirtfood Green Juice (kale, spinach, strawberries, green tea) + a small avocado slice on whole-wheat toast
- Lunch: Sirtfood Green Juice (celery, apple, green tea) + a serving of edamame pods
- Dinner: Turkey Meatballs

Day 4:

- Breakfast: Sirtfood Green Juice (kale, spinach, blueberries, green tea) + a small Greek yogurt with berries and a sprinkle of granola
- Lunch: Sirtfood Green Juice (celery, apple, lemon) + a chickpea salad sandwich on whole-wheat bread
- Dinner: Chicken Breast with Quinoa Salad (mixed greens, avocado) and a drizzle of balsamic vinegar

Day 5:

- Breakfast: Sirtfood Green Juice (spinach, parsley, apple, matcha) + a slice of whole-wheat toast with scrambled eggs and a side of spinach
- Lunch: Sirtfood Green Juice (kale, celery, pear, ginger) + a bowl of black bean soup with a side salad (lettuce, cucumber, tomato)
- Dinner: Tofu Scramble with Vegetables (onions, peppers) and a side of brown rice

Day 6:

- Breakfast: Sirtfood Green Juice (kale, spinach, strawberries, green tea) + a small handful of walnuts
- Lunch: Sirtfood Green Juice (celery, apple, lemon) + a tuna salad with mixed greens and a sprinkle of sunflower seeds
- Dinner: Salmon with Roasted Brussels Sprouts and a quinoa pilaf with herbs

Day 7:

- Breakfast: Sirtfood Green Juice (spinach, celery, blueberries, green tea) + a smoothie made with almond milk, berries, and a scoop of protein powder
- Lunch: Sirtfood Green Juice (kale, apple, green tea) + a lentil salad with chopped vegetables and a light vinaigrette

Sample 7-Day High Calorie Meal Plan (Around 1600-1800 kcal):

Day 1:

- Breakfast: Sirtfood Green Juice (kale, spinach, celery, apple, green tea) + a small handful of almonds and a cup of oatmeal with berries and nuts
- Lunch: Sirtfood Green Juice (kale, parsley, apple, lemon, matcha) + a grilled chicken breast with a side of roasted sweet potato and vegetables (broccoli, carrots)
- Dinner: Grilled Salmon with Quinoa Salad (mixed greens, avocado) and a drizzle of olive oil
- Snack: A small apple with a tablespoon of almond butter

Day 2:

- Breakfast: Sirtfood Green Juice (spinach, celery, pear, ginger) + ¼ cup rolled oats with berries, a sprinkle of chia seeds, and a dollop of Greek yogurt
- Lunch: Sirtfood Green Juice (kale, celery, apple, green tea) + a bowl of lentil soup with a slice of whole-wheat bread and a side salad (spinach, tomatoes)
- Dinner: Shrimp Stir-fry with Buckwheat Noodles and Vegetables (broccoli, carrots) with a drizzle of sesame oil
- Snack: A handful of mixed nuts and seeds

Day 3:

- Breakfast: Sirtfood Green Juice (kale, spinach, strawberries, green tea) + a small avocado slice on whole-wheat toast with a scrambled egg
- Lunch: Sirtfood Green Juice (celery, apple, green tea) + a serving of edamame pods with a small whole-wheat wrap filled with turkey and vegetables
- Dinner: Turkey Meatballs with Tomato Sauce and a side of brown rice and roasted asparagus
- Snack: A small pear with a square of dark chocolate (at least 70% cocoa)

Day 4:

- Breakfast: Sirtfood Green Juice (kale, spinach, blueberries, green tea) + a Greek yogurt parfait with berries, granola, and a drizzle of honey
- Lunch: Sirtfood Green Juice (celery, apple, lemon) + a chickpea salad sandwich on whole-wheat bread with a side of carrot sticks and hummus
- Dinner: Chicken Breast with roasted sweet potato wedges and a side of steamed green beans
- Snack: A small handful of dried fruit and a cup of green tea

Day 5:

- Breakfast: Sirtfood Green Juice (spinach, parsley, apple, matcha) + whole-wheat pancakes with berries and a sprinkle of walnuts
- Lunch: Sirtfood Green Juice (kale, celery, pear, ginger) + a bowl of black bean soup with a whole-wheat tortilla and a side salad (lettuce, cucumber, tomato)
- Dinner: Tofu Scramble with Vegetables (onions, peppers) served with a slice of whole-wheat toast and a side of brown rice with steamed broccoli
- Snack: A small cup of berries with a dollop of whipped cream

Day 6:

- Breakfast: Sirtfood Green Juice (kale, spinach, strawberries, green tea) + a scrambled egg with spinach and a slice of whole-wheat toast with avocado
- Lunch: Sirtfood Green Juice (celery, apple, lemon) + a tuna salad with mixed greens, a sprinkle of sunflower seeds, and a whole-wheat roll
- Dinner: Salmon with a side of quinoa pilaf with herbs and roasted Brussels sprouts
- Snack: A small apple with a tablespoon of natural peanut butter

Day 7:

- Breakfast: Sirtfood Green Juice (spinach, celery, blueberries, green tea) + a smoothie made with almond milk, berries, a scoop of protein powder, and a banana
- Lunch: Sirtfood Green Juice (kale, apple, green tea) + a lentil salad with chopped vegetables, a light vinaigrette, and a slice of whole-wheat bread
- Dinner: Shrimp scampi with whole-wheat pasta and a side of steamed asparagus
- Snack: A cup of herbal tea with a handful of air-popped popcorn

Chapter 5: Sample 14-Day Meal Plans for Phase 2

Day 1:

- Breakfast: Sirtfood Green Juice (kale, spinach, celery, apple, green tea) + a small bowl of Greek yogurt with berries and a sprinkle of chia seeds
- Lunch: Salad with grilled chicken breast (4 oz), mixed greens, avocado slices, balsamic vinaigrette
- Dinner: Salmon (6 oz) with roasted Brussels sprouts and quinoa (½ cup cooked)
- Sirtfood Green Juices: One in the morning and one in the afternoon

Day 2:

- Breakfast: Sirtfood Green Juice (spinach, celery, pear, ginger) + a slice of whole-wheat toast with scrambled eggs (2 eggs) and spinach
- Lunch: Lentil soup (1 cup) with a whole-wheat roll
- Dinner: Turkey meatballs (3 oz) with tomato sauce (½ cup) and a side of brown rice (½ cup cooked) and steamed broccoli
- Sirtfood Green Juices: One in the morning and one in the afternoon

Day 3:

- Breakfast: Sirtfood Green Juice (kale, spinach, strawberries, green tea) + a smoothie made with almond milk, berries, and a scoop of protein powder
- Lunch: Chickpea salad sandwich on whole-wheat bread with mixed greens (2 cups)
- Dinner: Tofu scramble with vegetables (onions, peppers) and a side of quinoa (½ cup cooked)
- Sirtfood Green Juices: One in the morning and one in the afternoon

Day 4:

- Breakfast: Sirtfood Green Juice (kale, parsley, apple, lemon, matcha) + a small bowl of rolled oats (½ cup dry) with berries and a sprinkle of nuts
- Lunch: Tuna salad (3 oz) with mixed greens (2 cups) and a whole-wheat cracker
- Dinner: Chicken breast (4 oz) with a side of roasted sweet potato (medium) and steamed green beans
- Sirtfood Green Juices: One in the morning and one in the afternoon

Day 5:

- Breakfast: Sirtfood Green Juice (spinach, celery, apple, green tea) + a slice of whole-wheat toast with avocado slices and a fried egg

- Lunch: Black bean soup (1 cup) with a side salad (mixed greens, tomatoes, cucumber)
- Dinner: Shrimp stir-fry with buckwheat noodles (½ cup cooked) and vegetables (broccoli, carrots)
- Sirtfood Green Juices: One in the morning and one in the afternoon

Day 6:

- Breakfast: Sirtfood Green Juice (kale, spinach, blueberries, green tea) + Greek yogurt parfait with berries, granola, and a drizzle of honey
- Lunch: Chicken salad sandwich on whole-wheat bread with mixed greens (2 cups)
- Dinner: Salmon (6 oz) with a side of quinoa pilaf with herbs (½ cup cooked) and roasted asparagus
- Sirtfood Green Juices: One in the morning and one in the afternoon

Day 7:

- Breakfast: Sirtfood Green Juice (spinach, celery, pear, ginger) + whole-wheat pancakes with berries and a sprinkle of walnuts
- Lunch: Lentil salad with chopped vegetables and a light vinaigrette (1 cup) with a slice of whole-wheat bread

- Dinner: Tofu scramble with vegetables (onions, peppers) served with a side of brown rice (½ cup cooked) and steamed broccoli
- Sirtfood Green Juices: One in the morning and one in the afternoon

Day 8:

- Breakfast: Sirtfood Green Juice (kale, parsley, apple, lemon, matcha) + a scrambled egg with spinach and a slice of whole-wheat toast with avocado
- Lunch: Tuna salad (3 oz) with a side salad (mixed greens, cucumber, tomato) and a whole-wheat wrap
- Dinner: Shrimp scampl with whole-wheat pasta (1 cup cooked) and a side of steamed asparagus
- Sirtfood Green Juices: One in the morning and one in the afternoon

Day 9:

- Breakfast: Sirtfood Green Juice (spinach, celery, blueberries, green tea) + a smoothie made with almond milk, berries, and a scoop of protein powder
- Lunch: Chickpea salad with mixed greens (2 cups) and a drizzle of olive oil and lemon dressing
- Dinner: Turkey chili (1 cup) with a side of brown rice (½ cup cooked) and a dollop of Greek yogurt

- Sirtfood Green Juices: One in the morning and one in the afternoon

Day 10:

- Breakfast: Sirtfood Green Juice (kale, spinach, strawberries, green tea) + a slice of whole-wheat toast with peanut butter (2 tablespoons)
- Lunch: Lentil soup (1 cup) with a side salad (mixed greens, carrots)
- Dinner: Salmon (6 oz) with roasted Brussels sprouts and quinoa (½ cup cooked)
- Sirtfood Green Juices: One in the morning and one in the afternoon

Day 11:

- Breakfast: Sirtfood Green Juice (spinach, celery, pear, ginger) + a bowl of rolled oats (½ cup dry) with sliced banana and a sprinkle of chia seeds
- Lunch: Chicken Caesar salad with grilled chicken breast (4 oz) and whole-wheat croutons (limited amount)
- Dinner: Tofu scramble with vegetables (onions, peppers) and a side of sweet potato (medium, baked)
- Sirtfood Green Juices: One in the morning and one in the afternoon

Day 12:

- Breakfast: Sirtfood Green Juice (kale, parsley, apple, lemon, matcha) + Greek yogurt parfait with berries and a sprinkle of granola
- Lunch: Black bean burger on a whole-wheat bun with mixed greens (2 cups) and a side of sweet potato fries (baked, limited portion)
- Dinner: Shrimp stir-fry with buckwheat noodles (½ cup cooked) and vegetables (broccoli, carrots)
- Sirtfood Green Juices: One in the morning and one in the afternoon

Day 13:

- Breakfast: Sirtfood Green Juice (spinach, celery, blueberries, green tea) + whole-wheat pancakes with a small amount of maple syrup and a sprinkle of nuts
- Lunch: Tuna salad sandwich on whole-wheat bread with mixed greens (2 cups) and a piece of fruit (apple, pear)
- Dinner: Chicken breast (4 oz) with a side of roasted vegetables (assorted) and quinoa (½ cup cooked)
- Sirtfood Green Juices: One in the morning and one in the afternoon

Day 14:

- Breakfast: Sirtfood Green Juice (kale, spinach, pear, ginger) + scrambled eggs (2 eggs) with spinach and a slice of whole-wheat toast
- Lunch: Lentil salad with chopped vegetables and a light vinaigrette (1 cup) with a whole-wheat roll
- Dinner: Salmon (6 oz) with a side of brown rice (½ cup cooked) and steamed asparagus
- Sirtfood Green Juices: One in the morning and one in the afternoon

Chapter 6: Customizing Your Sirtfood Meal Plan

The first step is to identify your individual needs. Consider factors like:

- Dietary Restrictions: Do you have allergies, intolerances, or follow a specific vegetarian, vegan, or gluten-free diet?
- Medical Conditions: Are there any underlying health conditions that require dietary adjustments? Consult a doctor or registered dietitian for guidance.
- Activity Level: Sedentary individuals may require fewer calories than someone who exercises regularly.
- Taste Preferences: Choose sirtfoods and recipes you enjoy to promote adherence to the plan.

Adapting the Sirtfood Approach:

Once you understand your needs, explore ways to personalize your sirtfood journey:

- Swapping Sirtfoods: Not a fan of kale? Explore other sirtfood greens like spinach or arugula. Experiment and find sirtfoods you enjoy incorporating into your meals and juices.
- Alternative Grains: If you're gluten-free, opt for sirtfood-friendly alternatives like quinoa, buckwheat, or brown rice flour.

- Plant-Based Proteins: Vegetarians and vegans can incorporate legumes, tofu, tempeh, or seitan as protein sources in place of meat.

- Healthy Fats: Include healthy fats like avocado, nuts, and seeds in moderation for satiety and nutrient absorption.

- Portion Control: Use measuring cups and spoons to ensure appropriate portion sizes, especially for higher-calorie sirtfoods like nuts and dark chocolate.

- Seasoning and Flavor: Don't be afraid to experiment with herbs, spices, and low-sugar condiments to add flavor to your meals without compromising the sirtfood principles.

Planning and Preparation:

Planning and preparation are essential for success. Here are some tips:

- Meal Prep: Dedicate time to prepping sirtfood ingredients like chopping vegetables or pre-cooking grains for the week ahead.

- Leftovers: Cook larger portions to have leftovers for lunch or quick meals throughout the day.

- Healthy Snacks: Have sirtfood-approved snacks like fruits, vegetables, nuts, or a small sirtfood green juice on hand to avoid unhealthy choices when hunger strikes.

- Read Food Labels: Be mindful of added sugars and choose sirtfood options with minimal processing whenever possible.

Chapter 7: Exercise for Women on the Sirtfood Diet

Regular exercise offers numerous benefits alongside the Sirtfood Diet, including:

- Increased Calorie Burning: Physical activity helps create a calorie deficit, essential for weight loss.

- Muscle Building: Building muscle mass can boost metabolism and promote fat burning even at rest.

- Improved Mood and Energy Levels: Exercise releases endorphins, which elevate mood and energy levels.

- Enhanced Bone Health: Weight-bearing exercises like strength training can help maintain strong bones.

- Reduced Risk of Chronic Diseases: Regular physical activity can lower the risk of heart disease, type 2 diabetes, and some cancers.

Finding Your Exercise Fit:

The ideal exercise program is one you enjoy and can stick with consistently. Here are some exercise recommendations for women on the Sirtfood Diet:

- Cardio: Aim for at least 150 minutes of moderate-intensity cardio or 75 minutes of vigorous-intensity cardio each week. Activities like brisk walking, running, swimming, cycling, or dancing are excellent options. Consider incorporating interval training for an extra metabolic boost.

- Strength Training: Include strength training exercises 2-3 times per week targeting major muscle groups. Bodyweight exercises, free weights, or resistance bands can be used to build muscle and improve bone density. Focus on proper form to maximize benefits and prevent injury.

- Low-Impact Activities: For beginners or those with joint issues, low-impact exercises like yoga, Pilates, or water aerobics offer a gentle yet effective way to get active. These activities improve flexibility, strength, and balance.

Sample Exercise Routine:

Monday: 30 minutes brisk walking + 20 minutes bodyweight strength training (squats, lunges, push-ups)

Tuesday: Rest or Active recovery (yoga, stretching)

Wednesday: 45 minutes swimming

Thursday: 20 minutes strength training (free weights or resistance bands) targeting upper body

Friday: 30 minutes cycling

Saturday: Rest or Active recovery (Pilates)

Sunday: Hike or explore a new outdoor activity

Chapter 8: Sleep and Stress Management

Adequate sleep is crucial for overall health and weight management. During sleep, the body undergoes vital repairs, regulates hormones, and consolidates memories. Here's how sleep impacts your Sirtfood journey:

- Hormonal Regulation: Sleep regulates hormones like leptin (promotes satiety) and ghrelin (increases hunger). Poor sleep disrupts this balance, potentially leading to increased cravings and overeating.
- Metabolism Boost: Sleep deprivation can negatively impact metabolism, making it harder to burn calories and lose weight.
- Sirtuin Activation: Research suggests that adequate sleep may promote sirtuin activity, the key mechanism behind the Sirtfood Diet's potential benefits.

How Much Sleep Do You Need?

Most adults require 7-8 hours of quality sleep per night. Here are some tips for improving your sleep hygiene:

- Establish a Sleep Schedule: Go to bed and wake up at consistent times, even on weekends, to regulate your body's natural sleep-wake cycle.

- Create a Relaxing Bedtime Routine: Wind down before bed with calming activities like reading, taking a warm bath, or light stretching. Avoid screens for at least an hour before sleep.

- Optimize Your Sleep Environment: Ensure your bedroom is dark, quiet, cool, and clutter-free to promote restful sleep.

- Limit Caffeine and Alcohol: Avoid excessive caffeine intake, especially in the afternoon and evening, as it can interfere with sleep.

- Regular Exercise: Regular physical activity can improve sleep quality, but avoid strenuous workouts close to bedtime.

Stress Management - Your Weight Loss Ally:

Chronic stress can hinder weight loss efforts. When stressed, the body produces cortisol, a hormone that promotes fat storage and increases cravings for sugary and unhealthy foods. Here's how stress management benefits your Sirtfood journey:

- Reduced Cortisol Levels: Effective stress management techniques can help regulate cortisol levels, promoting a more favorable hormonal environment for weight loss.

- Improved Food Choices: Stress can lead to unhealthy food choices. By managing stress, you can make more mindful dietary decisions aligned with the Sirtfood principles.

- Better Sleep Quality: Chronic stress can disrupt sleep. Stress management techniques can improve sleep quality, indirectly aiding weight management.

Stress Management Techniques:

Here are some strategies to manage stress and support your Sirtfood goals:

- Relaxation Techniques: Practice deep breathing exercises, mindfulness meditation, or progressive muscle relaxation to calm your mind and body.
- Physical Activity: Regular exercise is a great stress reliever. Aim for at least 30 minutes of moderate-intensity exercise most days of the week.
- Social Support: Connect with loved ones, engage in activities you enjoy, and seek professional help if needed.
- Healthy Habits: Prioritize self-care practices like getting enough sleep, eating a balanced diet, and staying hydrated. These habits contribute to overall well-being and stress resilience.

Conclusion: Unlocking Your Health Potential with Sirtfoods

Throughout this guide, you've explored the Sirtfood Diet, its core principles, and its potential to support weight management. You've learned about sirtfoods, their role in sirtuin activation, and the potential benefits for cellular health, metabolism, and overall well-being.

We've delved into practical aspects like creating personalized meal plans, incorporating sirtfoods into your diet, and navigating challenges that may arise. We've also emphasized the importance of sleep, stress management, and exercise for sustainable weight loss success.

The Sirtfood Diet is more than just a weight loss plan. It's a framework for establishing healthy habits that promote long-term well-being. By incorporating sirtfoods rich in nutrients and antioxidants, you're nourishing your body and potentially reducing the risk of chronic diseases. The focus on mindful eating, portion control, and a balanced diet lays the foundation for a healthy lifestyle that extends beyond the numbers on the scale.

As you move forward, remember these key takeaways:

Sirtfoods are Powerful Allies: Sirtfoods offer a delicious way to nourish your body and potentially activate sirtuins, promoting cellular health and metabolism.

Focus on Sustainability: Create a healthy lifestyle you can maintain for the long term. Prioritize mindful eating, portion control, and a balanced diet rich in sirtfoods.

- Embrace a Holistic Approach: Combine the Sirtfood Diet with regular exercise, adequate sleep, and stress management for optimal results.
- Celebrate Non-Scale Victories: Acknowledge improvements in energy levels, mood, sleep quality, and overall well-being, not just weight loss.
- Listen to Your Body: Pay attention to your hunger and fullness cues. Don't deprive yourself completely, and make adjustments as needed.

The Sirtfood journey is an ongoing exploration of healthy living. Use this guide as a springboard to continue learning, experimenting with sirtfoods, and refining your approach to healthy eating and well-being. Remember, you are capable of achieving your health goals and unlocking your full potential.

www.ingramcontent.com/pod-product-compliance
Lightning Source LLC
Chambersburg PA
CBHW051656250726
48653CB00007B/2692